We Can Be Responsible!

WE STAY HEALTHY

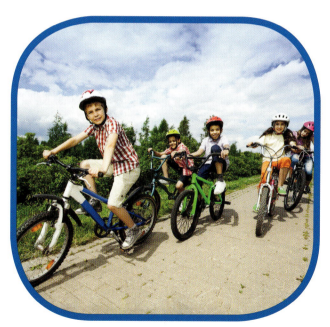

By Lynda Arnéz

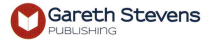

Please visit our website, www.garethstevens.com. For a free color catalog of all our high-quality books, call toll free 1-800-542-2595 or fax 1-877-542-2596.

Library of Congress Cataloging-in-Publication Data

Names: Arnéz, Lynda, author.
Title: We stay healthy / Lynda Arnéz.
Description: New York : Gareth Stevens Publishing, [2020] | Series: We can be responsible! | Includes index.
Identifiers: LCCN 2018038743| ISBN 9781538239261 (pbk.) | ISBN 9781538239285 (library bound) | ISBN 9781538239278 (6 pack)
Subjects: LCSH: Health–Juvenile literature.
Classification: LCC RA777 .A763 2020 | DDC 613–dc23
LC record available at https://lccn.loc.gov/2018038743

First Edition

Published in 2020 by
Gareth Stevens Publishing
111 East 14th Street, Suite 349
New York, NY 10003

Copyright © 2020 Gareth Stevens Publishing

Editor: Kristen Nelson
Designer: Sarah Liddell

Photo credits: Cover, p. 1 Sergey Novikov/Shutterstock.com; p. 5 Anna Nahabed/Shutterstock.com; pp. 7, 24 (broccoli) Kateholms/Shutterstock.com; p. 9 Lyubov Kobyakova/Shutterstock.com; p. 11 picturepartners/Shutterstock.com; p. 13 Africa Studio/Shutterstock.com; p. 15 Pressmaster/Shutterstock.com; pp. 17, 24 (bike) JGA/Shutterstock.com; p. 19 Hafiez Razali/Shutterstock.com; pp. 21, 23 Robert Kneschke/Shutterstock.com.

All rights reserved. No part of this book may be reproduced in any form without permission in writing from the publisher, except by a reviewer.

Printed in the United States of America

CPSIA compliance information: Batch #CS19GS: For further information contact Gareth Stevens, New York, New York at 1-800-542-2595.

Contents

Many Ways. 4

Good Food 6

Staying Clean 10

Be Active and Rest 14

Together! 20

Words to Know 24

Index. 24

There are lots of ways
we can stay healthy!

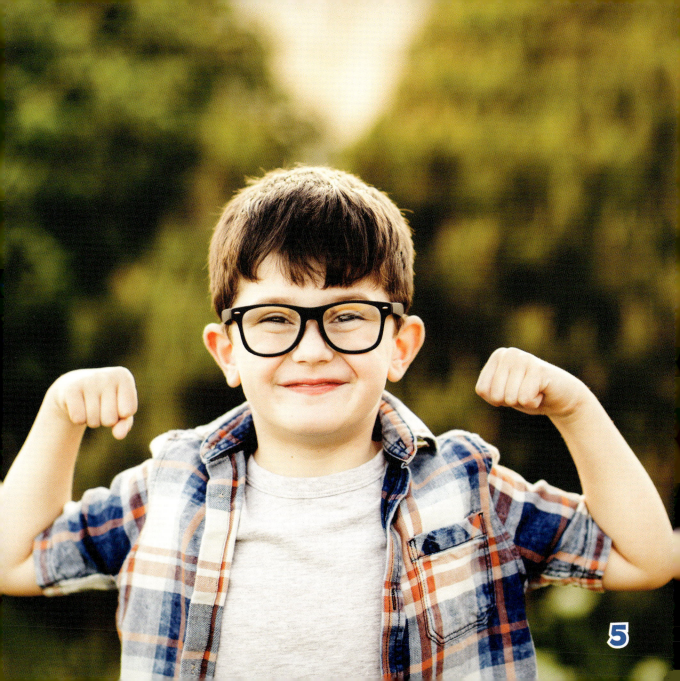

Maury eats vegetables.
He loves broccoli!

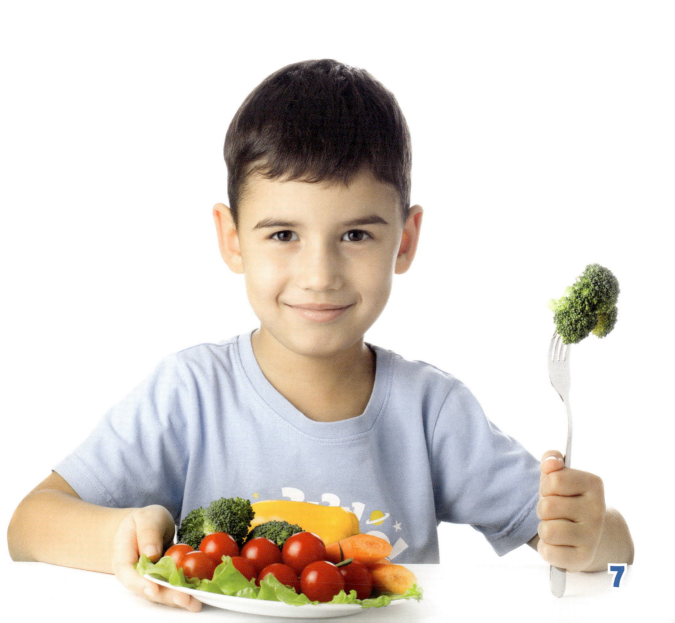

Caroline likes fruit.
She eats an apple!

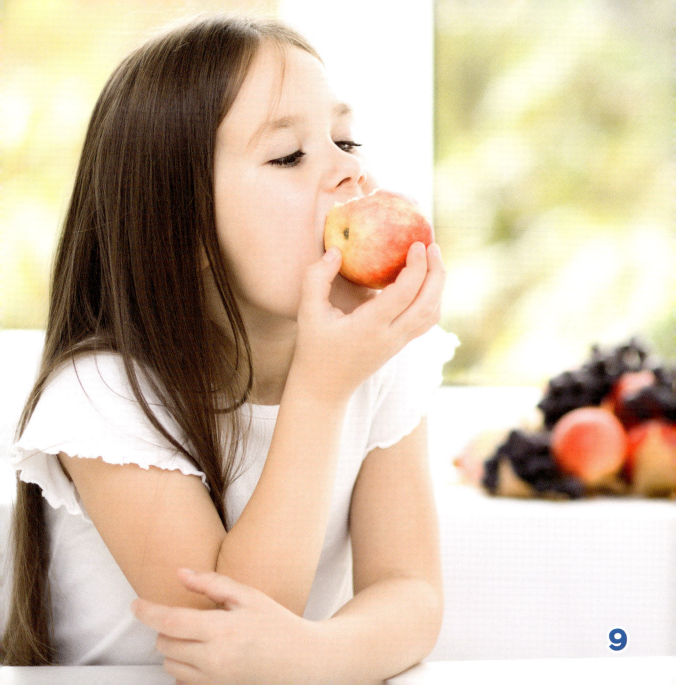

Taylor washes his hands.
It helps him not get sick!

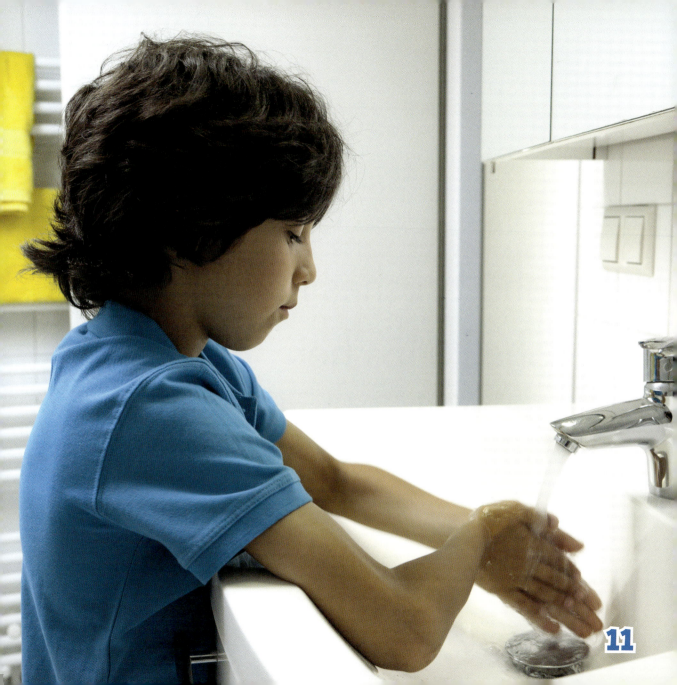

Isha brushes her teeth.
She keeps her
mouth healthy!

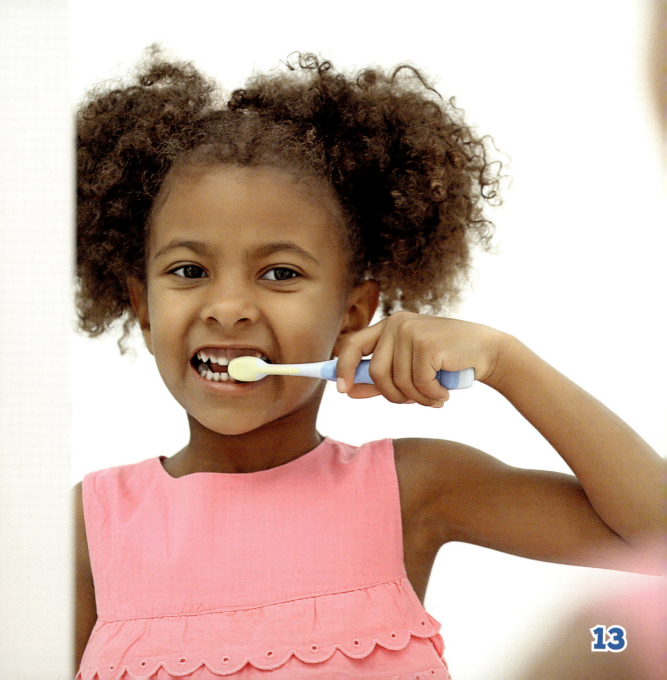

Exercise makes our body strong. Sports are fun!

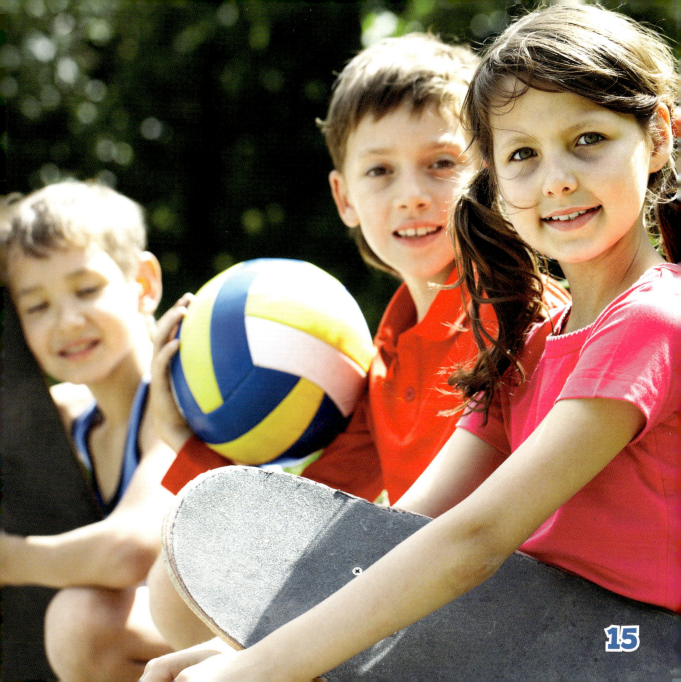

Suri loves to ride her bike.

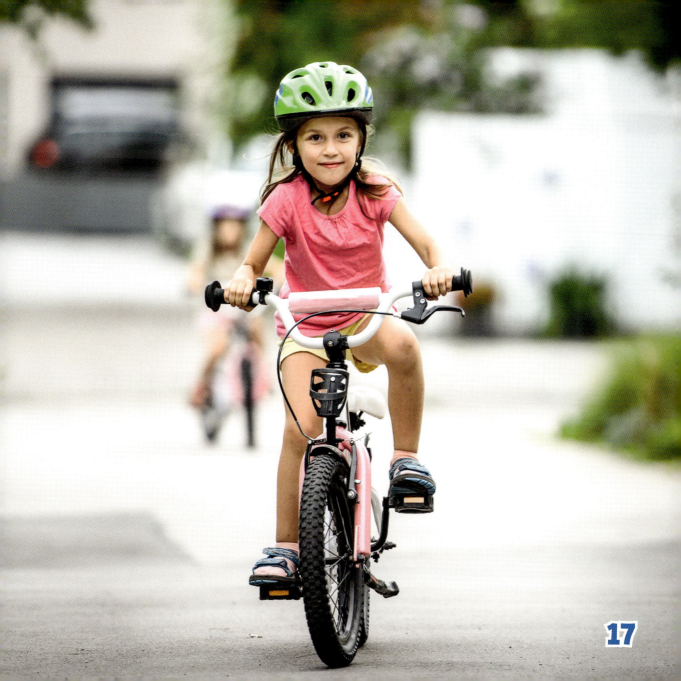

Sleep keeps us healthy!
John goes to bed on time.

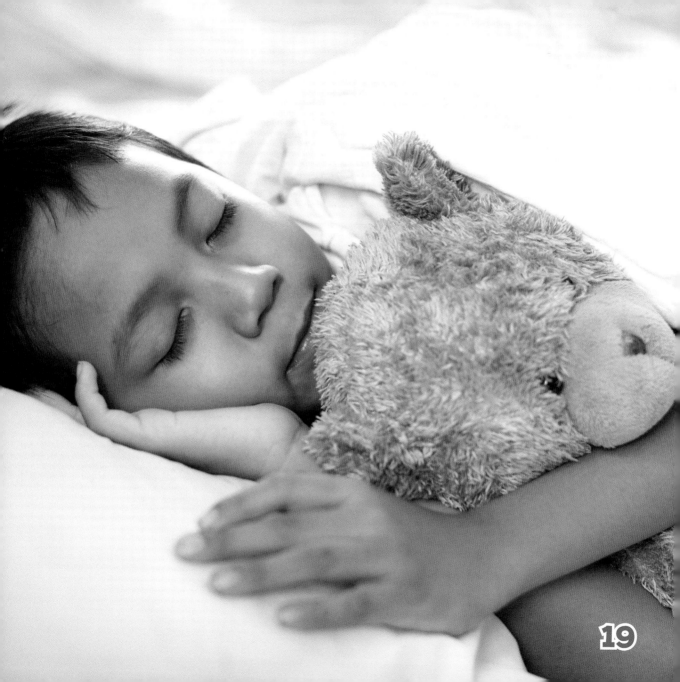

Having friends helps us stay healthy!

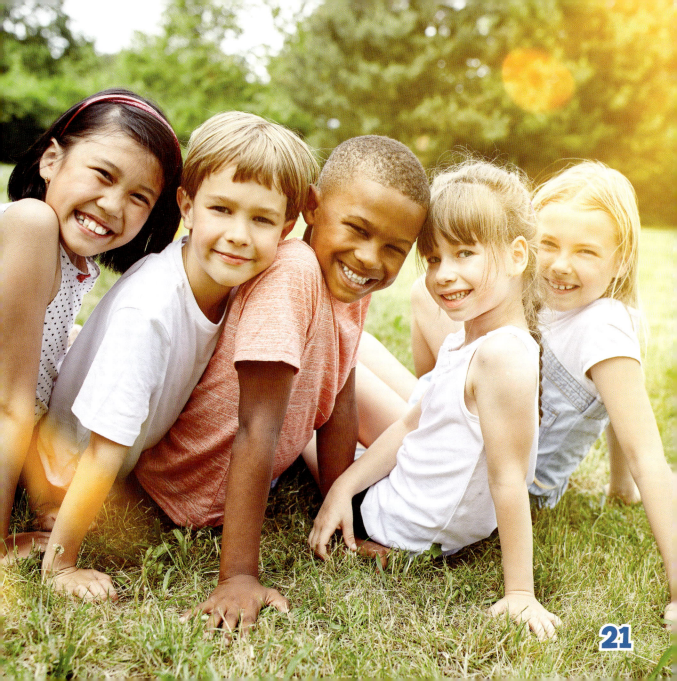

How do you stay healthy?

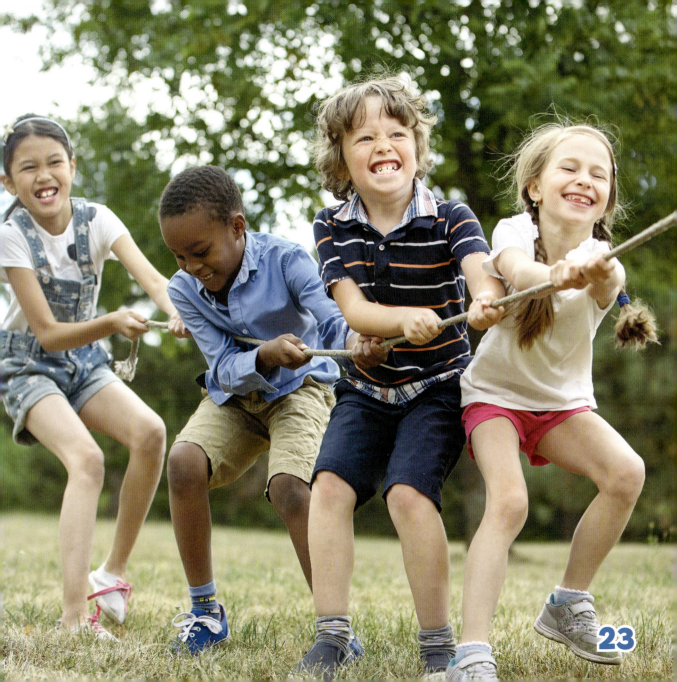

Words to Know

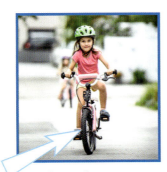
bike

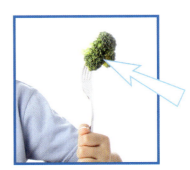
broccoli

Index

exercise 14

fruit 8

sleep 18

vegetables 6